FIRST TIME DAD

Your Role Before Baby Arrives

Ian McGivern

Copyright © 2022 Ian McGivern.

ASIN: B09Q98PQTD

Table of Contents

INTRODUCTION

You're going to be a first-time dad, Congratulations! You will soon learn that there is no handbook for being a perfect father. Every baby is different, and every situation is unique, so you will just have to wing it as you go along. That said, there are some things that all dads should know about the three trimesters of their child's life.

After reading this book, you will be able to prepare yourself for the trials and tribulations of fatherhood. It is perfect for first time fathers who have just been told the news or have just gotten over the shock. It explains what she is going through and gives tips on how you can support her during this exciting but trying time in your lives.

Pregnancy is divided into three trimesters, each with its own unique set of challenges and rewards.

Your book is written with 4 main parts:

First Trimester: 0 – 12 Weeks

Second Trimester: 12 – 24 Weeks

Third Trimester: 24 – 40 Weeks

Birth: Surviving the first 6 Weeks

For each of these you will learn what to expect and how you can help your partner and survive the roller coaster journey you are about to embark on.

No bs (or as much as I could keep out) has made it into this book. Updates are provided for each trimester with how your baby is growing, what mum is going through and what you can and should be doing.

Each section also finishes off with a Top 10 Things what NOT TO SAY.

'Cause face it… boys will be boys.

So, strap in and let's go!

HELP HER FEEL BETTER (FIRST TRIMESTER)

Conception - 12 Weeks

Hey, you're going to be a dad! And you're probably freaking out because you have no idea what that means. First off: What's normal? For starters, woman can go through all sorts of emotions during pregnancy: You might find her crying one minute and laughing the next. She might get cranky -- then again, so will you when those nights start coming around where neither of you can sleep because your little one just kicked up a storm in there or made themself comfortable in some other uncomfortable place.

Being pregnant is a rollercoaster ride for all three of you, and I cannot emphasize it enough when I say that IT'S OKAY TO BE UNCOMFORTABLE. It is totally normal to have morning sickness where she throws up every time that she smells food cooking (and don't even think about entering the kitchen uninvited). It is normal to gain 2-4 pounds during the first trimester (and about a pound a week for the rest of the pregnancy. It's also normal for her ankles to swell up like two grapefruits. If you have not figured it out already, none of this is pleasant -- but this too shall pass (in 9 months or so).

So, what can you do?

For starters: Be supportive. Do not give her a hard time when she's puking or wants to lie down in the middle of watching TV. Sometimes the best thing you can do is just be there and let her know you have her back, even if it means bringing her a bucket or holding her hair back.

Do research so you know what questions to ask your doctor -- and do not be afraid to call, email or text with your concerns. It's better to get an answer and feel stupid than it is to not ask at all and do something that could end up causing irreparable damage (or pain).

Be understanding when she says 'no.' This goes double for the late stages of pregnancy when her body is changing daily and she's trying to get comfortable enough for both.

Do not give her a hard time when she gets emotional either. Her hormones have been going wild and, as a result, so has she -- do not be surprised if she cries at a commercial for a dishwashing detergent or something equally random. It might not always make sense, but just go with it.

Take the initiative and help around the house. She might not want to get up from her comfy spot on the couch, so if you see stuff piling up in the sink or hear an empty milk jug calling your name -- take care of it!

What else? Let her know she is beautiful when she doesn't feel like it. Take care of the pets. Do the dishes without being asked (seriously, you'll be glad that you did). When in doubt, just ask yourself "WWGD?" -- What Would Gentleman Do?

How Is Baby Developing During The First Trimester?

The first trimester is the time when a baby's body and brain are developing.

During this period, a baby will grow from an embryo to a fetus. This development includes the formation of organs, muscles, bones, and skin.

Your partner might start to feel pregnant symptoms during the first trimester such as fatigue or morning sickness.

Development also involves establishing connections between nerve cells in the brain called synapses. These connections allow messages to be sent back and forth between different parts of the brain so that they can learn new things like how to crawl or walk for example.

It's also the time when you, the dad-to-be, begin to make a transition from being a partner in crime with your wife to becoming a parent.

Here are some changes you can expect to see in both your wife and yourself...

How Is Mommy Developing During The First Trimester?

The first trimester brings many body changes. Baby will need lots of nutrients, so the mother's appetite has increased to keep up with the demands of becoming a mommy. She may have frequent headaches, fatigue, heartburn, constipation, nausea, vomiting, and the feeling of being bloated.

Headaches are often caused by hormonal changes in her body. You can help relieve your partner's headaches by giving her a massage. She will appreciate this gesture!

Constipation is also common because hormones slow down digestion, so she doesn't have to go to the bathroom as often.

Nausea and vomiting are symptoms of pregnancy known as morning sickness. It is more likely to happen in the early months of your baby bump adventure, and it will most likely go away by week 14 or 15.

You can help soothe your wife's stomach by cooking her favorite meal or buying her a gift that shows you care!

1) Her Sleeping Patterns May Change

During the first trimester, your partner may have difficulty sleeping because her hormones are changing constantly. She may suffer from insomnia or night-time waking due to pregnancy symptoms such as indigestion, cramping, back pain, or heartburn.

You can help your partner through this tough time by buying her some scented candles, organizing the bedroom or cooking (or ordering) her a tasty meal.

2) Nausea or Morning Sickness

Nausea is common in the first trimester of pregnancy and usually begins around week 6 after conception. The nausea can be accompanied by vomiting since morning sickness typically occurs during the morning.

If the nausea is bad, your wife may vomit more than once a day.

There are several things you can do to help ease her nausea:

Make sure she drinks enough water and eats dry foods like toast or crackers between meals. Keep your home environment smelling fresh and clean by using a scented candle or essential oil. Make her some home-made chicken soup (Google a recipe if you don't have one!)

3) Pregnancy Cravings and Aversions

Hormonal changes can affect which foods your partner desires as well as those she does not want to eat because of morning sickness, nausea, food aversion, growing baby bump or heartburn.

You can help your partner find relief by making her favorite food or dessert, getting take-out or catering for dinner, and/or doing the grocery shopping.

4) Body Temperature Changes

During pregnancy, mom might have higher body temperature

sometimes, which is caused by an increase in blood flow to the surface of the skin and a decrease in the ability to perspire.

This helps her body regulate itself and keep both baby and mommy safe, but it can lead to overheating during warm weather or even at home if she has too many layers of clothing on.

You could buy your partner a cooling scarf or tank top, set up a fan by her bedside, and give her some ice packs to place on her neck and forehead when she feels hot.

5) Her Personal Grooming Habits May Change

During the first trimester your partner may not feel like herself or up to styling her hair, putting makeup on, or fixing a cute outfit that makes her look great. She might be too tired to shower or brush her hair.

As a partner, do not push her to do her hair and makeup because it might not be a priority to her anymore! Make sure she eats well and gets enough sleep so she can look after herself the best way possible.

6) Your Partner ~~May~~ WILL Experience Mood Swings

Hormonal changes during the first trimester of pregnancy can cause mood swings. Your partner may feel like she is on an emotional rollercoaster, and everything is either amazing or extremely difficult.

This is normal and it might last until the end of the typical 40-week pregnancy term, but it also depends on how your partner was before she became pregnant.

You can help her cope with mood swings by finding out the cause of her emotions so you both know what to do or not to do. You could also try to make time for activities that you used to enjoy together, playing games, and watching movies at home, and reminding her that this is probably just a short phase in her pregnancy.

7) Your Partner May Suddenly Have Darkening of the Areolas

The darkening of the areolas—the pigmentation around your partner's nipples—is a normal change that sometimes occurs during pregnancy as her body prepares for breastfeeding after baby is born.

You can support your partner by simply accepting her as she is and admiring how beautiful she looks, even if her breasts are larger or look different.

8) Body Hair Growth May Increase

The body hair growth is caused by the same hormone responsible for pregnancy symptoms like nausea and vomiting. You can support your partner by shaving her legs and underarms, moisturizing her skin with a rich lotion or oil, and finding out if there is anything else you can do to make her feel more comfortable.

9) Your Partner May Experience Heartburn

Heartburn—a burning sensation in the chest caused by stomach acid coming up from the stomach to the throat. It is another common pregnancy symptom that can take place during all three trimesters.

Your partner may experience heartburn as a mild discomfort, but it can also be painful and disrupt her sleep. You could offer to bring her some water or an antacid and let her know you are there for her if she needs anything to make the pain go away.

10) Your Partner May Be Constipated

Common pregnancy symptoms can include constipation, but it is also one of the most common digestive problems that pregnant women experience, especially during the third trimester.

You can help her by encouraging her to drink plenty of water and eat foods like bananas, prunes, or raisins to help keep her digestive system moving.

What To Expect As A First-Time Dad During The First Trimester

The first three months of your baby's life is the most fragile, and as a father to be play your role during these 3 months. There have been great changes that happened not just in your spouse but also in you as a man. You might feel surprised and scared thinking how your life would be as a father.

Well, you must take into consideration that the first three months is just a period where a strong bond is being built between you and your baby, thus making you feel protective of both yourself and your spouse from now on. It is during the 1st trimester where doubts might start to creep in your mind. These doubts might be wondering if you are doing everything right or worrying too much.

Take note that it is quite common for first time dads to feel this way, so don't worry as here are some things you might feel during the first trimester period.

The feeling of worry and lack of confidence starts to come into your mind during this time because you worry too much that things could go wrong with the baby, your spouse or yourself. You might blame yourself for not being ready right away, which is very normal as first timers usually feel this way even if they really do want to have a baby.

The feeling of excitement and responsibility also begin to sink in as you start to love this new life inside your spouse's womb, even if it is too early for you to feel such emotions yet. You will begin to share responsibilities with your partner by being there through all the things that she needs help with during this period.

The first trimester is also like a honeymoon phase where you will enjoy the feeling of making plans for your future child's arrival and discuss about baby names. You might feel this nervous, excited yet extremely happy feeling during these times that you cannot wait to see your new family.

Your role here, and throughout the pregnancy, is one of support.

How To Help Her Deal With Morning Sickness And Fatigue

Some moms-to-be love the idea of morning sickness because it means they are pregnant.

Others would rather eat a bag full of rat poison than throw up their breakfast every day for months on end. If your partner is in this camp - and she very well may be - you might need to step in and take care of her.

There are a few things you can do to help your wife out during the first trimester:

- Offer to take care of the household chores while she rests
- Bring her breakfast in bed and keep it light. No greasy bacon or sausage for her! Unless she insists, and face it buddy... you have no choice :-)
- Get her fresh fruit, vegetables, and plenty of water. Dehydration can make nausea worse
- Bring her ice chips or popsicles to help with the nausea
- If she's feeling up to it, take her on walks or for light bike rides. Exercise can help reduce fatigue
- Give her a hug (or ten) and tell her you love her

How To Help Your Partner Prioritize Her Emotions (Because Lord Knows I Needed Help!)

It's hard for pregnant women to prioritize their emotions, because so many different things are going on.

She's probably feeling overwhelmed, anxious, and maybe even a little bit scared. This is normal!

- Encourage her to talk about her feelings with you or other friends/family members. Keeping them bottled up will only make them worse.
- Help her stay organized and on top of the household chores (or better yet, do them for her!)
- If she wants to talk about it, listen and be supportive. Try not to interrupt or jump in with advice unless she asks for it!
- Avoid telling her that you understand how she feels (even if you think you do). No one can truly know how another person is feeling, so let her tell you about it.

- Ask what you can do to make her feel better. This is the best way to show support and love for your partner and mother of your baby! The more specific, the better (for example: "Can I make dinner tonight?" or "Do you want me to take over laundry duty today?")

Things That Made Me Happy During The First Trimester (And Things That Didn't)

Whether this is your first time around or not, the first trimester of a pregnancy can be a crazy time. You may be feeling a mix of emotions – from happiness and anticipation to fear and anxiety. Here are some things that made me happy during my first trimester (and some that didn't).

Take it from me, you'll get through it!

Things That Made Me Happy

- Feeling the baby move for the first time
- Finding out it was a girl (Technically that happened in the Second Trimester, but hey, I needed a win here)
- Getting her nursery ready
- Planning her birthday party (Yea yea, I know - far away, but hey!)

Things That Didn't Make Me (or more specifically my wife) Happy

- Morning sickness – ugh!
- Tiredness and fatigue – She felt like she couldn't do anything
- Mood swings – one minute she was happy, the next she wanted to cry

- Heartburn – It felt like my wife's stomach hurt all of the time
- Insatiable hunger - I swear she ate constantly!

Things That Helped Us Get Through It All (And Things We Wish Someone Had Told Us)

This is by no means a complete list, but here are some things that helped me get through the first trimester with my wife.

- Keep doing what you're already doing – being supportive and caring for your spouse is so important!
- Get out of the house together when she has an energy spike (and make sure to give her lots of hugs)
- Find a new hobby or activity that you can do together to take your mind off things.
- Give her space when she needs it, but don't forget about her! Sometimes just being there is enough for someone who's feeling down.

Things We Wish Someone Had Told Us

That the first trimester would be over SOONER than we thought.

AND that the tiredness would go away eventually. It didn't feel like it but trust me – day by day she got a little more energy!

Your First Doctor's Appointment

At your first doctor's appointment, you'll probably have the ultrasound. The ultrasound is important because this will be where they take the measurements to see your baby's gestational age.

Keep in mind that this information can change, so do not worry if you are unsure about the accuracy of it.

You'll also learn how big your child is at any given point (in centimeters). This will help you determine their approximate weight and other vital statistics like lengths and head circumference. None of this will be useful in the future when you want to buy them their first outfit!

The Ultrasound is also where they'll measure your child's nuchal translucency, which gives an idea for potential birth defects or chromosomal abnormalities. This information may not have any impact on whether you are able to have the child, but it is important to be aware of.

At your first appointment, you will also hear your baby's heartbeat for the first time! It's an amazing experience. The sound of that little heart beating is truly incredible.

Tips For Surviving Your First Doctors Appointment

- Go with your partner - she'll need you there.
- Bring a notepad and take notes. You will want to remember everything the doctor says!
- Ask questions, lots of them. The doctors are happy to answer anything you want to know.
- Take pictures or videos if you're allowed (check with your doctor first). This is such a special moment to share with friends and family.

When Is The Right Time To Tell People About Your

Pregnancy?

You might be thinking, "Should I wait until the first trimester is over?" or "What if someone tells me not to say anything?"

You've probably already told most of the people closest to you, but maybe you're still waiting for that perfect moment. When should you tell other people, like co-workers or distant relatives?

Here are some ideas:

Family and close friends

It's usually best to tell people closest to you as soon as possible after you confirm the pregnancy. The reason for this is so they can support you during your early months, which are often the most difficult ones.

Work Associates

Some women feel uncomfortable telling their co-workers about their pregnancies until they're past their first trimester, while others prefer to tell colleagues right away, so they have the support of people at work.

This is a conversation you need to have with your partner. If you decide to wait until after your first trimester, be sure not to share anything with your or her co-workers because it could lead to them accidentally revealing that information to others before you are ready.

Relatives and Friends

For people who are more distant, it can be a challenge to decide when and whether to share something so personal. Here's what you need to think about:

If these people will be involved in your pregnancy or expect to receive updates about the baby such as invitations to the birth or baby shower, consider telling them sooner rather than later. If you know they won't be involved, then you can decide when to share the news.

The Bottom Line

There is no "right" time to tell people about your pregnancy. Each pregnancy and each situation is different, so only you and your partner can decide when it's best to let people know or if you'd rather not say anything at all.

Top 10 Things You Should Not Say During The First Trimester

Many new fathers will not understand how difficult it is for a woman to carry a baby. In fact, you wouldn't even know what's happening with her if she doesn't tell you. For that reason (and because I stepped in some landmines), I have put together this list of things that you should NOT say during the first trimester:

1) "I hear morning sickness is worse at night."

I know this was meant to be helpful but the last thing she needs while hugging the toilet is someone trying to brighten her day. So instead of saying this phrase, learn what helps (massage and peppermint tea worked for us).

2) "You can do it!"

Fellow new dads might be saying this. There's nothing wrong with giving your partner encouragement during her darkest hour. But remember, she is not physically able to bear the load of your unborn baby. Just say, "I'm here for you."

3) "You should take a pregnancy test."

Unless she brings it up first (which rarely happens), new dads will be tempted to ask if she took one yet. Don't do it! She'll decide when she's ready.

4) "Do you need anything?"

Again, she'll tell you when she needs something. Making suggestions is fine but don't force her to ask for anything. The only thing this question does is make the expectant mother feel guilty that she's not doing more to help herself in a time of crisis.

5) "Let me know if I can help."

Please don't say this. Instead, DO something! You are her husband or partner, and she needs you to be physically there for her instead of asking again and again if there's anything you can do. She already knows that. And please stop saying "I'm sorry" when you have nothing to apologize for.

6) "I hope it's a boy."

Maybe she does too, but you need to let her have this one. If your partner is having a gender reveal party, then that's another story. Personally, gender didn't matter for me. I was blessed with a daughter and would have loved my baby regardless of gender.

7) "Did you eat anything?"

Your partner is at the point where her body is turning inward and supporting your baby for nine months. She probably lost her appetite too. So even if she says, "No," it's probably a lie. Let her keep this one up and feed herself as much as she needs or wants.

8) "Is it time yet?"

Even if she's in her third trimester, don't say this! It makes her feel like she's carrying a watermelon instead of your child. She will let you know when the baby is coming. Trust me on that one.

9) "Can I drive you somewhere?"

Let it go, buddy! That's another one she won't appreciate. Driving around is the last thing on her mind. She likely feels insecure about her body and doesn't want to be seen by everyone until after she delivers. Just give her your arm if you are walking somewhere together or stay close by in case, she needs to lean on you.

10) "Is this normal?"

When she says, "I'm tired," it doesn't matter if your other pregnant mom friends are still working out three times a week. Tell her that you love her and then organize her some naps or anything else she needs. Mom to be needs to know that her partner will be there for her physically, emotionally, and spiritually.

> Don't forget to say "I love you" every day... even if she's driving you up a wall. That's what she needs to hear most of all!

SPOIL AND PAMPER HER (SECOND TRIMESTER)

Week 12 - 24

The second trimester is a crucial time for you baby's development. It's when the fetus will develop their fingers and toes, as well as internal organs such as their lungs and liver.

Your partner may feel as though your baby is growing at a quick pace now. In addition to all of this, she'll finally get some energy back! As for you, it may seem like your baby is becoming more active now. You'll feel them move around a lot at this stage!

Changes You Can Expect

Your partner's body will be changing quite a bit during the second trimester. Her belly will grow bigger, and she might have morning sickness again (though not as bad). In addition to that, her skin may start breaking out and she might feel hungrier than ever before.

The Second Trimester Is A Great Time To Start Preparing For The Baby.

You can start buying clothes and toys, as well as making a list of things you'll need for the hospital.

I've got some suggestions on the essentials later in this chapter.

How Can I Help My Partner?

The best way to help her during the second trimester is by being supportive and understanding. Listen to her when she wants to talk and be there for her when she needs it.

In addition to this, you can make her feel special by planning a date night every week. Get out of the house and spend some time together!

Baby Is Growing!

Mum will start to feel baby move around more and you may even be able to hear the heartbeat. You'll also start to see more of your baby's features as they grow.

Your child now measures over three inches from crown to rump and weighs almost an ounce, about as much as a large lemon. Their taste buds are formed, but their lungs aren't ready for breathing air. They can make a fist, open their mouth, move their tongue side-to-side and recoil like a startled turtle.

Baby's brain is growing rapidly. Seeing and hearing are developing too, but baby can't tell what they see and hear from one moment to the next. They recognize your voice now, especially when you sing! By 26 weeks your baby's eyes can sense light.

Now that your baby's liver is producing bile, their digestive system is more able to process wastes. The digestive system itself consists of two parts: the gastrointestinal tract (oesophagus, stomach, and intestines) and the liver, pancreas, and gallbladder. This stage, the gastrointestinal tract starts to contract in a pattern like breathing in and out. The intestines begin to absorb fats and proteins which they need to function properly.

The nervous system is hard at work too! Baby's brain is continuing its rapid growth. The neural tube along baby's back is closing. This protects the spinal cord and keeps baby's backbone from fusing together. The neural tube also forms brain stem, cerebellum, cerebral cortex, and the retina of your child's eye in this stage of development.

Your partner will be feeling a mix of emotions – from happiness and anticipation to fear and anxiety.

Here are some things that made me happy during the second trimester (and some that didn't). Take it from me, you'll get through it!

Things That Made Me Happy

- Feeling our baby move for the first time
- Finding out the gender of our baby (Got Confirmation)
- Watching my wife's belly grow

Things That Made Me Less Happy

The fear and anxiety that came with knowing we were going to be parents soon.

How Mommy-To-Be Is Developing During The Second Trimester

Her body has gone through a lot of changes and your baby is becoming increasingly active as they get ready for the outside world. You and your partner may feel like you are getting used to it all, but so far this pregnancy has probably been nothing compared to what's coming. Second trimester brings even more changes, and you may feel like you and your partner are busier than ever.

Second trimester, which starts at about 14 weeks, is when many of the final changes happen before birth. Around week 18, your baby will drop down lower into your partner's pelvis. This is called lightening because it lightens the load on your lungs! It's about time, and it feels good.

At 20 weeks, your baby is considered full-term, and your partner might begin to feel really big or notice that her clothes aren't fitting as well as they used to. This is normal, because most of the weight gain in pregnancy happens during this trimester (about 1/2 pound to a pound per week).

Your partner's uterus is about the size of a basketball right now, and she'll begin to feel many of the discomforts of the second trimester. She may have more tender breasts or feel nauseous or tired all the time. As fatigue sets in, encourage her to rest as much as possible.

She's probably also feeling other big changes in her body as well. She may notice more hair on her legs or underarms, and she may sweat a lot more as the pores in those areas open. More hair on her face is normal too because of increased levels of hormones. She may feel bloated, especially in the afternoon, and she'll probably need to use the bathroom more often-up to six times a day!

It's becoming more difficult for your partner to find comfortable sleeping positions. Most women start to sleep on their sides at this stage because it feels better when they're up all night with back pain. It's also good for your baby, who is now more than 10 inches long and weighs over 12 ounces! Your partner may be able to feel your baby move every day now, but if she hasn't yet, don't worry. Even though movements are stronger, they may still be too small for her to feel.

What You As A Dad Can Expect During The Second Trimester

During the second trimester of pregnancy your partner is going to be experiencing some physical changes that may bring on discomfort and aches. She will also experience emotional changes as her body begins to prepare for birth. There are many things that your partner can expect to experience during this time, I have listed a few of the most common below:

Second Trimester Physical Changes

Your partner's body is changing in many ways. All these changes are complicated processes that involve the uterus growing, breasts becoming more sensitive, hormones flooding multiple systems and much more. The best thing you can do for your partner at this time is to be supportive and understanding.

Her breasts will be changing and may become very tender, you cannot really miss them now that they are growing. Her nipples are becoming more sensitive as well, she may even leak some fluid from her breasts that is called colostrum. This occurs because her breasts are beginning to produce milk. You can help your partner by massaging and washing them gently, beside the tenderness they will also be much larger than usual.

Your partner's belly is now big enough for you to place your hand on the outside and feel the fetus moving around. This is a fun experience that I highly recommend sharing with your partner.

As her belly grows, she may find it difficult to stand, walk and sit comfortably. Sometimes a pillow behind her back or under her belly can help her maintain a more comfortable position.

Your partner may gain some weight during the second trimester; however it is all about balance and moderation. You do not want her to eat unhealthy foods just because she is pregnant, but also keep in mind that you should be encouraging her to eat healthy foods by making them for her and having fun food experiences together.

Second Trimester Emotional Changes

When your partner's belly gets big enough, she will begin to feel the baby moving around inside of her. This is great because it allows you to communicate with your baby and her to feel them as well. Once the baby starts kicking, she may gain a feeling of protectiveness over her unborn child and strong feelings of love.

Your partner's emotions are much more sensitive during this time. She could be incredibly happy one minute and then extremely sad the next. This is all because her hormones are changing rapidly, however try to offer words of encouragement when she is feeling down.

It may be difficult for your partner to concentrate on daily tasks, keep in mind that this is due to the changes in her hormones. She may not want to get up early and go for a walk, she may even get angry sometimes. Try and do simple things with her like taking a bath together or going for a ride in the car.

RENT A TRAILER AND GO BUY DIAPERS

You can start stocking up on diapers and other supplies. You do not want to be caught unprepared when the baby is born. For us, this meant renting a trailer and heading out to buy diapers! Not really, but I wish we did.

Is It Time To Start Buying Clothes?

You can start buying clothes for your baby, but don't go too crazy. Babies grow out of clothes quickly, so you may not need as many as you think.

Your partner will also start to show more now, so it might be a good time to take some maternity pictures!

Adjustments To Your Lifestyle

The second trimester is a good time to adjust your lifestyle. If you're not used to an active lifestyle, now might be the time to start (or at least exercise more). You'll need all of that energy for chasing after the baby!

Some other things you can do are:

- Keep riskier hobbies like skydiving and cliff jumping to a minimum
- Drive more carefully – you don't want anything bad happening!
- Get or update your life insurance
- Get or update your will

Planning Baby's Room

You can start thinking about what you want your nursery to look like. This includes the colors, theme, and decorations.

It's also a good time to start thinking about what kind of crib you want, as well as other furniture.

Common furniture include:

- Changing table
- Dresser (with a changing pad on top)
- Side Table for Diaper Cream and Other Supplies

Renting A Trailer and Going Out To Buy Diapers! I know I've brought up those diapers already, but man, you're gonna need a crap load (pun intended).

What About The Name?

This is a big question that many couples face during the second trimester. Start discussing names and see if there are any that both of you like.

Don't be in too much of a rush. My wife blurted out, very randomly I may add "Alexa" from the shower one morning.

Top 10 Things Not To Say During The Second Trimester

1) "I Miss the way things Used to Be"

This is a tough one. After finally coming to terms with the fact that you should know what you are doing by now and your partner should not be crying every day because she maybe should have thought about children before she got pregnant…you might think it's time to start bringing up the good old days again. This is a huge mistake! Your partner is still hormonal and more importantly she is carrying your child inside of her. She has no idea if it might be a boy or a girl, if this will be the kid that loves sports or hates them. All she knows for sure that at some point you WILL be telling her how much better everything was before and that's what triggers these episodes. Don't do it.

2) "Are You Sure Everything is Normal?"

During the first trimester, either the morning sickness or the hormones had your partner convinced everything was not normal. She would say things like "Is our baby going to be born with six toes?" and you would reassure her that everything was fine, and babies were not usually born with extra toes. Well guess what? Morning sickness has faded and so have the hormones, but there is definitely something wrong this time.

This leads to your partner calling you in tears because she just heard that babies are not normally born without kidneys or some other essential organ. If you thought for one second that she was being ridiculous before, now is the time to let her know that you think she might be right.

3) "Do We Need a Car Seat?"

Your partner spent enough time researching car seats during the first trimester. She knows what she wants. Keep in mind that some prams come with a detachable car seat.

4) "You Really Should Buy Some Baby Clothes"

This is not the time for presents. Your partner has no idea if this baby will be a boy or girl, so she wants to save everything until you know. However, there are some essentials that an infant needs. The best solution here would be taking your partner shopping for essentials like diapers and wipes. If you really want to buy clothes, then some neutral colors, like yellow, could work.

5) "You Should Try and Have a Nap"

Yes, your partner is tired. Very Tired. But the couch does not look comfortable, and she doesn't think she can sleep anyway so why bother trying? It is like telling someone to relax in a dentist chair right before they get a root canal. Don't do it!

6) "Can we go out to eat?"

Your partner is tired and wants to sleep. She also does not feel great most of the time so eating at home is just easier. You have responsibilities now! If you want that steak, then cook it at home or just do what your partner suggests which is to pick up some food on your way home. You are tired too!

7)"I'm sorry, but I can't help you with the dishes right now."

Your partner is feeling a little better now, so she finally has the energy to do some housework. It's likely that she'll want to start with something really easy like doing the dishes or maybe folding your laundry from last week. This is not the time for you to say you have too many emails and spreadsheets to sort through on your laptop. She needs your help.

8) "You look so tired!"

Your partner may still have those dark circles under her eyes from being so tired. However, telling her she looks as bad as a zombie who is about to be shot by the main character of a horror film is not going to make her feel any better.

9) "Stop crying, it's not that bad."

Your partner cried a lot during the first trimester. She cried because she was sick, she cried because of morning sickness, and she probably even cried at work because it was just too overwhelming. Now that your partner is feeling better there's a good chance that she might start crying again...and no matter what you do don't tell her to stop!

10) "How much weight have you gained this week?"

Your partner is super aware of her weight and how it's changing day by day. She is also very conscious about what she eats at every meal, so you don't have to remind her that she needs to go on a diet. This might be the time when you need to comment on how good she looks!

MAKE HER FEEL COMFORTABLE (THIRD TRIMESTER)

Week 24 - 40

Congratulations! You're almost there!

The Third Trimester is the most exciting part of pregnancy. Your baby has now grown to over a pound (about 1.3 pounds at 24 weeks) and has a fully developed body that can move around freely.

What You can Expect during this Trimester

Your baby will continue to grow. You'll start to see more of the features that make your child unique, and you may be able to feel their feet pushing against your wife's belly.

The Third Trimester is an exciting time for both parents. You'll be getting closer to meeting your child, and they will start to look more like a human being.

Enjoy it!

What can you do during this exciting time to make it easier on yourself and your family?
- Get the nursery ready (furniture, paint, theme)
- Pack bags for after the birth of your child

A.k.a. "The Hospital Bag" or "Birth Bag" this is what you take with to where your partner is going to deliver. Ps. Be sure to memorize all routes to the hospital and traffic congestion density at certain times of the day :-)

Sample contents of the Bag:
- Phone charger
- Camera
- Snacks and drinks for mom and dad
- Your partner's going to want her own pillow
- Toiletries (toothbrush, toothpaste, shampoo, soap)
- Entertainment (books, magazines, headphones)

Tips For First Time Dads During The Third Trimester

When my wife told me that our baby was the size of a grapefruit, I was like, "What do you expect me to do with that information?" Well, now that you're in the home stretch of her pregnancy—the third trimester—I thought I would share some more tips. If you're like I was and have no clue what you're doing, these pointers should come in handy.

- Relax! Your wife is going to need your support more than

ever
- Prepare for the birth – try watching some videos and educating yourself on what might happen
- Get as much sleep at night as you can because it's only going to get worse from here (you'll be up all hours of the night with a crying baby)
- Try not to stress about money. You might feel like you're spending way too much on diapers, wipes and clothing but remember that the baby is only going to be small for a short time
- Attend parental classes with your partner

Prenatal Classes – Why And What To Expect

Also known as antenatal classes, prenatal classes give expectant parents an opportunity to gain experience about the birthing process and what you can expect when your child is born. They often include topics such as health, safety, and hygiene within pregnancy; breathing and relaxation techniques; information about possible labour stages, breathing and discomfort management. It is especially important classes for new parents to attend so you can prepare yourself and become more aware about pregnancy, baby's birth, and baby care.

You can take antenatal classes when your baby is between 30-34 weeks in the womb (beginning of the third trimester). You could start antenatal classes before 28 weeks but leaving it for later means it will be fresh in you and your partner's memory.

Many hospitals offer them for free or at low cost because attending these classes is an important part of prenatal care. There are other places where you can take them too, like community centres and home study groups. However, it is best to check with your doctor first so they can advise you where to go.

You are not obligated to attend antenatal classes, but they have a positive impact on your birth experience.

Typical things you will learn are what happens during labour, breathing techniques to use when in pain, what you need to take to the hospital with you, how to know when it is time for you and your partner to go to the hospital.

You also get a chance to ask questions about pregnancy concerns or just broad questions that are bothering you. It's good to attend these classes with your partner, so you can know what to expect on your baby's birth day.

Antenatal classes are very informative and useful, they will help you feel less nervous about the birth day.

Prenatal classes can also be stressful (or helpful, depending on how you look at it). Most of them are held in groups which means you will be surrounded by other people who are pregnant. So, you can feel a bit uncomfortable because everybody is listening to your problems and experiences about pregnancy. Chances are many in the room are going through the same thing.

You should go for prenatal classes if you want to know what to expect during labor or improve your knowledge about childbirth or baby care. They are very useful and will prepare you for the birth day so attend them. This is where I gained most my knowledge.

Stages Of Labor And Delivery

No one can really prepare you for what's to come. But, in case you're curious (or just need to know what kind of horrors to expect), I'm going to walk you through the different stages of labor and delivery. Buckle up because it's about to get real!

What to expect during labor and delivery:

- Early labor – this can last for a few hours or a few days. Contractions will be mild to moderate and may be irregular. This is the time to relax and get some rest
- Active labor – contractions will become stronger, more regular, and closer together. You'll want to head to the hospital at this point
- Transition – this is the time when your partner will be most likely to say things like, "I can't do it" and "Why did I think having a baby was a clever idea?"

Pain Relief Options

Once your partner is in active labor, she will be given pain relief options. And trust me, she is most likely going to want something!

Here are the most common types of pain relief:

- Epidural – a shot that is given through the spine and numbs the entire lower half of the body

- Spinal Block – a single injection into the lower back that numbs the nerves from the waist down

- Nitrous Oxide – a gas mask offers your partner some relief by calming her body and reducing pain

- IV Sedation – this is also known as "twilight sleep," which results in a state of semiconsciousness. Your partner will not remember anything after she receives it

- Natural Childbirth – some women choose to go without pain relief and rely on breathing exercises and relaxation techniques

Tips For Getting Through The Stages Of Labor And Delivery

As you prepare for the arrival of your little one, you will inevitably have a lot of questions. One of the most important things to know is what to expect during labor and delivery. Here's a guide to help you through it all.

- Keep your partner comfortable. This is her time to shine, so take care of any needs she might have
- Remain calm no matter what happens – you're the rock that will keep your family together during this crazy time! Staying calm will be so helpful for your partner!
- Make sure you have everything ready to go before baby arrives. This includes diapers, wipes, clothes, and a place for baby to sleep

Top 10 Things Not To Say To Your Wife During Labor And Delivery

It's your first time as a dad, and there's so much you want to say to your partner during labor and delivery. Unfortunately, not all those things are wise or helpful. Here's my list of the top 10 things NOT to say to her during labor and delivery.

1) "I don't know how you're doing this."

Believe me, she doesn't either!

2) "You're not doing it right."

Huge red flag here. Just don't go there. She's the expert on how to birth her baby, and she doesn't need any unsolicited advice from you. Keep your thoughts – and words – positive until she asks for your opinion!

3) "Stop screaming/crying/yelling/yodelling or whatever it is that you're doing."

Many women choose to vocalize during labor and delivery. If your wife is one of them, encourage her through her noises by saying "You're doing great," or something similar. She's probably feeling a lot of pain, and it helps when you tell her that you know it's hard but that she's doing swell.

4) "When is this going to be over?"

Many women labor and deliver for hours and hours before the baby actually arrives. If your wife is busy pushing a baby out of her, don't distract her by asking when she'll be finished. It won't help. You'll know when it's over!

5) "Is that what I think it is?"

Your partner knows exactly what she's making, thanks.

6) "I hope our baby looks like me."

Now may not be the best time to mention how much you want a paternity test.

7) "How much longer do you think it'll be?"

Although a legitimate question, asking it will only put your partner on the defensive and sour her mood – not to mention make both of you crazy. Ask yourself this: how long can I go without knowing? If your answer is "Not longer than two minutes," you may want to direct your question to the nearest nurse.

8) "I can't manage this."

A woman's ability to give birth is so much more impressive than yours, so it's best not to put her abilities down by saying something like this. Instead, refer back to advice #1 and keep your comments (and facial expressions) positive.

9) "I need a break."

She's birthing your child right now, so don't make her feel like she has to take care of you too. When you're tired or overwhelmed, go outside for some fresh air and then come back into the room with your game face on.

10) "I'm so glad that's over!"

It may seem like it to you, but your partner is still working hard – even if she doesn't look like she is. Remember that what seems like an eternity to you feels like just a few seconds to her!

BE HELPFUL AND PROTECTIVE

(Birth and First Days)

Welcome to parenthood! As a new dad, you are probably feeling a range of emotions - elation, exhaustion, terror, and many more. One thing is for sure - you want to be helpful and protective of your new baby. Here are some tips to make the first few days go as smoothly as possible.

Enjoy this crazy ride!

Day 0+ For Your Baby

Your baby will need to stay in the hospital for a few days, even if all seems well. But don't worry – your child will be given a thorough examination by the doctors and nurses before going back home!

Day 0+ For You

You are a parent now. Enjoy that role while it lasts, because soon you'll find yourself doing all of the things, they say about parenting in those old cliches – "It's a 24-hour job," "Your life is never going to be the same again" and so on...

No matter how prepared you think you are for labor and delivery, nothing can really prepare you for the real thing. But that's okay! If you know what kind of horrors to expect. Buckle up because it's about to get real!

- Early labor – this is the time when your partner will start to experience some mild contractions. This can last anywhere from a few hours to a few days
- Active labor – contractions will become stronger, more regular, and closer together. You will want to head to the hospital at this point
- Transition – this is the time when your partner will be at her most uncomfortable. It is the shortest stage of labor, lasting only about one hour
- Delivery – this is when you will meet your new child! Welcome to parenthood!

After Delivery

If everything goes according to plan, this will be a time of joy as you welcome your new child into the world! Your first moments with your child will be a blur, but make sure to take some time to just relax and enjoy this special moment. However, if your partner experiences any problems after delivery – such as excessive bleeding or infection – she may need to stay in the hospital for a while.

After giving birth, most women feel tired and sore. Have plenty of pillows and blankets on hand to make her comfortable. Also make sure you have a car seat ready to take your baby home in. You will need to take your baby to the hospital for a check-up within the first few days after delivery.

If your partner is breastfeeding, make sure she has a breast pump and plenty of milk storage bags. Pumping will help her produce more milk.

5 Things You'll Regret Doing The Day Your Baby Is Born

- Not sleeping when you have the chance
- Skipping out on a shower
- Forgoing breakfast or lunch
- Neglecting to take pictures of your baby in those first few hours
- Leaving the hospital before you're supposed to. If something goes wrong, you won't be able to return as easy!

Making sure that you have everything ready to go before your baby arrives. This includes diapers, wipes, clothes, and a place for your child to sleep are all important factors in making sure you have an easy time during this crazy time!

Bringing Baby Home - What To Expect In Those First Few Weeks

- Your baby will need to eat every two to three hours, around the clock. This means that you will probably be up a lot in the middle of the night
- Babies this age usually sleeps for 16-20 hours per day.

Try to take advantage of nap times whenever possible
- Expect your house to be dirty and messy for a while. It is hard to keep up with everything when you're also trying to take care of your new child
- If it is difficult to get out of the house, expect that this will be where you will spend most of your time in those first couple weeks!

A Survival Guide To Sleep Deprivation

- Make sure to stock up on coffee and other caffeinated beverages. You will need them!
- Get as much help from family and friends if you can. Having an extra set of hands will make the sleepless nights so much easier for both you and your partner
  - If baby is fussy, try walking around with them or allowing them to take a bath. You can also try swaddling, but make sure you leave the arms loose
- The best thing that worked for us was breastfeeding! When my wife put our baby on her breast, she would usually fall asleep in minutes

Having an infant will be one of the most difficult yet rewarding experiences of your life. Just remember to take it one day at a time and do not be afraid to ask for help when you need it!

The Roller Coaster You'll Experience Post Birth

- Not knowing how to hold the baby, and worrying you will break them
- Wondering why your child won't stop crying! When will they start sleeping through the night?

The first thing that happens after your partner gives birth is that you meet your new little one. You may or may not have an idea of what to expect, but it's likely you won't know what true love feels like until this moment (to someone else, other than your partner, of course).

Babies change so much in the first few weeks that they might not feel familiar to you anymore.

When your baby starts sleeping through the night is different for everyone! You'll just have to wait and see when your little one has had enough of being up all the time.

Get ready to feel like a chicken with its head cut off - you will be constantly running around trying to take care of everything.

When your child reaches their first birthday, it will seem like they have been part of the family forever. Time flies!

The bond between a father and his new child is something truly special. Just remember to take it slow and be patient with yourself as you figure out this new life!

You'll lose your temper at some point or another.

Having a newborn baby can be one of the most difficult things you will do in your lifetime, but also one of the best experiences you will ever go through. Prepare yourself for the roller coaster ride of emotions that come with this new chapter in your life!

You might also feel guilty about not loving them right away.

Newborn babies are a handful, but they're so worth it. Just keep reminding yourself why you decided to have one and be patient as you figure out how to be a new parent!

You might feel like you're doing everything wrong, and that no one is there to help you.

Be sure to take care of yourself and your significant other as best possible - this will make the transition into parenthood much easier on everyone involved. Prepare yourself for sleepless nights, lacklustre days, and a complete lack of time for yourself!

But you'll find your groove again soon enough.

Get ready to feel like a zombie during the day and always be tired. There is no such thing as staying up late anymore - because babies don't sleep in!

Tips For Enjoying The First 6 Weeks With Your Newborn

Stock up on groceries and prepare for a lot of take out.

Plan to do nothing but stay at home for the first few weeks post birth, if possible.

Help your partner out as much as possible - it will make the days go by so much faster!

The first six weeks after having a baby are an adjustment - but it is also a time to just relax and enjoy your new little one. Here are some tips to make the most of this special time!

- Make sure your partner gets as much rest as possible in between feedings
- Don't be afraid to ask for help from friends and family, you'll need it!
- Enlist the help of a postpartum doula if you can afford it!

They are worth every penny

Top 10 Things Not To Say To Your Partner When You Get Home After Labor And Delivery.

There are a few things you should know about the first few weeks after your baby is born. First and foremost, DO NOT SAY ANY OF THE FOLLOWING TO YOUR PARTNER.

Happy wife, happy life!

1) "What's for dinner?"

This is the first question you ask? Really?! The woman just spent hours in labor, pushing out a watermelon size baby through her wooha! And that is what you're worried about? You can head to the shop and grab some chow mein on your way home - I am sure even the hospital canteen is better than her cooking now.

2) "Why are you crying?"

Well, quite frankly, because I just pushed out a baby out of me woo hoo. She is emotional, maybe she's got the hormones flowing through her system - who knows? But give her some time to settle down and do not be so insensitive to ask this question!

3) "Why are you so tired?"

She is tired because... well, I give you 3 guesses :-) And even with all the adrenaline in her system, she's still exhausted. And do not say that it's just because she was up all night.

4) "Can I go back to work now?"

Sure, just take the baby with you. While you are at it, can you get me a latte too?

5) "I'm going to take a shower and then we should go out for dinner."

You don't think cooking for her, or takeaways will be a better option?

6) "I'm really tired."

Really? Because it looks like you are fresh as a daisy. And thanks for taking over while I nap.

7) "You should put on some weight."

The postpartum diet is not a good time to insult her.

8) "I'm going to watch something on TV."

And leave me with the kid? Way to make a new mom feel welcome home!

9) "Show me what you bought today"

Didn't you just ask her what's for dinner?

10) "I'm going to sleep"

You are lucky she even lets you sleep in the same bed! Good luck tomorrow night when it is diaper change time!

But seriously, you just received the greatest gift that life can offer. It is up to you to take care of your partner and baby... And make sure to avoid saying anything from the "Top 10 What Not to Say" lists.

And do not forget that every day will
only get easier :-) All the best!

Our Baby Is Home, Fed And Breathing... What Now?

Keep a look out for my follow-up books, where you get even more great, no bs advice.

* 9 7 9 8 4 0 2 3 0 7 8 3 4 *